Disclaimer

The advice and claims made about specific superfoods on or through this book have not been evaluated by the United States Food and Drug Administration or the Canadian Food and Drug Administration and are not approved to diagnose, treat, cure or prevent disease. The information provided in this book is for informational purposes only and is to be followed at your own risk. It is not intended as a substitute for advice from your physician or other health care professional.

You should consult with a health care professional before starting any diet, exercise or supplementation program, before taking any medication, or if you have or suspect you might have a health problem. We cannot be held responsible for typographical errors or product formulation changes. Please consult with your own physician or health care practitioner regarding the information provided in this book and especially before using any advice provided in this book.

Please visit my informative website for more on Superfoods.

thesuperfoodsbook.com

Dedicated to my children; Selena, Molly, Lucy and Thomas.

Superfoods – What are superfoods?

The newspapers, magazines, and television are filled with news about superfoods, but what are they and why should you care?

Foods become classified as superfoods when they possess traits which provide greater health benefits than other foods. This can be in the form of high amounts of vitamins and minerals, but often other factors play an even larger role. Many of the foods we currently classify as **superfoods are extremely high in antioxidants** which appear to play an essential role in helping our bodies fight off disease, reduce the risks of cardiovascular problems, and even stop the growth of cancer.

Improved Energy and Moods with Superfoods

The role of disease control may be important but for me there is an even more important reason to eat superfoods. They provide me with increased levels of energy, better mood control, an increased libido, and an overall feeling of wellness. Would you consider changing your eating habits slightly in order to change your life?

Some superfoods fall into one other category. **Super Foods help people who are overweight to lose weight easily.** Can you picture being able to enjoy delicious substitutes for the foods which have produced your obesity and that all you to lose weight at the same time? It is possible! You might be shocked to discover this even includes eating certain types of chocolate, delicious yogurt desserts, and other foods which are amazing. I enjoy drinking an ice cold green smoothie whenever I want with the knowledge it is not going to increase my weight. Do you want to start enjoying food and getting health benefits at the same time?

The Simplicity of Changing to Superfoods will astound you

Let us look at a quick example of how easy it is to start transforming your life with superfoods. How do you start your morning? For many of us our morning starts off with a donut, a cup of coffee with creamer and sugar, plus a bowl of cold cereal laced with sugar. Can you see a problem? The meal is packed with sugar, fats, and almost zero nutrition. Let us look at an easy alternative which is just as delicious.

Try starting your morning with a cup of black tea with a touch of raw honey to give it a slightly sweet taste. Then you can add a bowl of yogurt kefir with some blueberries and a few slivered almonds tossed in. If you are feeling really hungry and adventurous add a buckwheat pancake to your breakfast. You suddenly have a breakfast which is using six different superfoods which are high in vitamins, minerals, antioxidants, and dozens of other trace nutrients. The difference in your energy levels is tremendous.

With that old way of eating you have a spike of energy to start the day and usually by mid-morning you feel lazy, lethargic, and ready for a nap. Concentration levels plummet as your energy levels drop-off since you chose to eat a breakfast packed with sugar.

With your **new way of eating by adding superfoods you have energy which lasts**. The buckwheat, blueberries, kefir, and almonds all release energy must slower. You have high amounts of dietary fiber which aids in slowing sugar absorption. You discover you are awake, alert, and focused all the way to lunch. This is where the next challenge usually occurs in our lives.

The Afternoon Energy Drop Starts with Your Mouth

What do you eat for lunch? When I watch most people head out to lunch they run to their favorite fast food restaurant or race to eat the sandwich they packed in the morning. It is usually washed down with a soft drink dense in sugar. Then as a reward for surviving the morning they eat a cookie, candy bar, or other sweet dessert to finish up the meal. Does that sound like your lunch? How do you feel in an hour, two hours, or just before work finishes for the day? I will bet you feel awful. Your energy is gone. You want to get home. You can hardly think.

Your life can be so different if you just change your eating habits slightly. You can have energy which lasts until supper. You can have mental alertness which will shock you. You can feel alive, excited, and motivated all day long. **Your body and mind respond to the fuel they receive, with superfood fuel they go into overdrive**. Let us take a look at an alternative lunch which would empower you.

Let us start off your lunch with large salad which has a mix of fresh spinach leaves and romaine lettuce. You add a light dressing made from extra virgin olive oil, vinegar, and a few spices. I like a little bit of a spicy flavor so I usually add a little cayenne and hot peppers to my dressing. Add a few sprouts to the salad and some toasted barley and cashews. For dessert eat a piece of kiwifruit. If you want a really refreshing beverage drink a tall glass of iced green tea. If you insist on it being sweet add a touch of honey.

Once again we have created a meal which contains numerous superfoods. In this case we have 11 separate superfoods listed. Eating this meal is guaranteed to give you more energy, higher cognitive ability, and better health than the other meal. What is going to shock you is this second meal tastes better, too. You will never understand how good fresh foods taste until you give this a try.

Change Your Life with Superfoods

What is even more important is what is beginning to happen inside of your body. The improved energy levels are not temporary. As you keep eating with a high emphasis on superfoods and quality you will notice you feel energetic almost constantly. You will experience less frequent colds, allergy symptoms, and you can be fighting against cancer, heart disease, and even the onset of Alzheimer's disease.

I want to ask you a very serious question. If you could start to enjoy eating more, save money, and improve your health dramatically would you do it? This is not an idle promise. The **benefits of superfoods are backed with scientific and medical research which is growing in volume**

daily. It is time for you to reclaim your life and it all starts with a simple decision to begin including superfoods in your diet. It is time for us to explore some of the great superfoods you can add to your diet.

55 Nutrient Rich Superfoods

Acai

- 100 grams organic unsweetened berry puree
- Calories – 80
- Carbohydrates – 6g
- Protein – 8.1g
- Total Fat – 32.5
- Dietary Fiber – 44.2g
- Calcium – 260mg
- Iron – 4.4mg
- Vitamin A – 1002U
- Aspartic, Glutamic, and Amino Acids – 7.59% of weight

The Acai Berry has become one of the world's most recognized superfoods due to massive marketing efforts in recent years. The acai berry is packed with anothocyanins, proanthcyanidins, and flavonoids. These phytochemicals are high in antioxidant properties and provide anti-inflammatory properties also. The powerful antioxidant properties aid in the reduction of cell membrane damage and DNA degradation which can be caused be free radicals in the body.

Acai berry can be found in many different forms. Health food stores commonly carry fresh acai berries, acai juice, and the freeze dried powder. You can find acai puree' available in many gourmet shops and health food stores, also. The berries and puree' can be used to make shakes, fruit salads, added to yogurt, or even eaten fresh. The freeze dried powder is best used in shakes which are well blended.

The most enjoyable form of the acai berry is the fresh berries and puree' which maintain the most flavors. Fresh berries are a wonderful addition to a bowl of oatmeal with your breakfast. Most acai berry juices are blended with other fruit juices. Take time to check the label carefully to make sure of the actual acai berry percentage.

Adding just a small amount of acai to your diet on a daily basis can help increase your overall health due to the high antioxidant and anti-inflammatory properties. Try a variety of ways to enjoy this amazing little berry. One added way to eat the acai fruit is to follow the lead of the natives of the Amazon forest where the berry originates by adding the fruit to tapioca. Acai berries can play an important role in improving your health while providing you with a delicious treat.

Almonds

- 25 nuts raw
- Calories – 170
- Carbohydrates – 5g
- Fats – 15g
- Dietary Fiber – 4g
- Protein – 6g
- Calcium – 12% Daily Value
- Iron – 21% Daily Value
- Vitamin E – 80% Daily Value

Ready for a tasty treat from the nut family? Almonds are one of my favorite snacks and garnishes for other dishes and thankfully it is another of the highly nutritious superfoods. Almonds provide you with tremendous amounts of energy in a tiny package. A handful of almonds weighing only 100 grams give you 581 calories of power packed energy, but more importantly it is a slow release source of energy instead of the rapid blast of energy you get from foods high in sugar content.

Almonds must be consumed in moderation due to the high fat content but these are not necessarily unhealthy fats. One of primary fats in almonds is responsible for lowering LDL cholesterol and blood lipid levels which can improve your cardiovascular system. Almonds are one of the best sources of natural vitamin E you can find. That handful of almonds gives you nearly 2 times the daily requirements of vitamin E. Vitamin E contributes to better skin condition, improved libido, and plays a role in improving mental and nervous system responses.

When you start adding in the high amounts of B vitamins, minerals, and protein it is no surprise this superfood is a highly recommended snack by dieticians, doctors, and nutritionists. My favorite way to eat almonds is also the easiest. I like to keep a package of dry roasted almonds ready to snack on at any moment. Grabbing a small handful of these nuts is great way to get that added energy and nutrition you need. I enjoy using thinly sliced almonds in my salads, in vegetable dishes, and mixed with my yogurt or kefir. This is one superfood you will never struggle to enjoy since they are simply delicious.

Almond milk

- 250 ml – 8 fl oz
- Calories = 70
- Total Carbohydrates = 10g
- Cholesterol = 0g
- Sodium = 0g
- Total Fat = 3g
- Saturated Fat = 0g
- Dietary Fiber = 0g
- Sugars = 0g
- Protein = 3g

The awesome almond is packed with healthy oils and full of natural antioxidants, they help to lower total cholesterol and thus are good for your heart. Almonds are also good for protein. About 50-60 grams of protein a day is good for an adult. Raw almonds are best, once pasteurized they lose much of their nutritional value. A handful of raw almonds eaten daily will give you your natural daily vitamin E quota. Vitamin E is a powerful anti-aging agent and essential for brain-body coordination. Most westerners have a vitamin E deficiency. Like all superfood nuts, almonds should be purchased fresh and raw. Label them with the date and store in your fridge in airtight containers for up to 9 months. If you have to roast them do so at a temperature of 150 degrees for 20 minutes. If you roast above 170 degrees you will lose the health benefits they provide.

Almond Milk Recipe

Soak 1 cup of raw Almonds overnight. Drain water and discard. Now blend 3 cups of fresh water with the Almonds and a teaspoon of natural Vanilla extract until smoothly blended. Now strain the entire mixture. Cheesecloth is good or a fine strainer. Keep fresh in the fridge for up to 4 days. Use in green smoothies. Almond milk can replace a lot of recipes that require cow's milk and Vegans use it often. It is also a good replacement for Soy milk. The strained pulp is great for adding to steel cut oats with natural yoghurt and Blueberries at breakfast. Almond milk can be sweetened with Stevia although some people dislike the licorice aftertaste. Agave nectar is also an option but high in calories. If you are not a vegan then raw honey makes a good sweetener. Vanilla extract and dates are also used for sweetening. Remember this recipe also applies to Brazil nuts, cashew nuts, and hazel nuts too.

Apples

- 125g – average size apple
- Calories = 50

- Total Carbohydrates = 17g
- Cholesterol = 0g
- Sodium = 0g
- Total Fat = 0g
- Saturated Fat = 0g
- Dietary Fiber = 3g
- Sugars = 13g
- Protein = 0g

An apple a day keeps more than the doctor away. One large apple equals 30% of your daily fiber needs. Combine an apple with a banana, berries and crushed ice in a meal replacement smoothie daily and you will get most of your daily fiber needs and knock off a few hundred bad calories. All of that fiber helps to fill up your stomach. Apples are crammed with antioxidants, have lots of vitamins, phytonutrients and potassium. Always eat the skin with the flesh as most of the nutritional value is concentrated in the skin. Apple skin contains four times more antioxidant potency than the entire flesh of the apple. Apples are good for the heart and the lungs.

Arugula

- 2 cups
- Calories = 8
- Total Carbohydrates = 1.5g
- Cholesterol = 0g
- Sodium = 0g
- Total Fat = 0.5g
- Saturated Fat = 0g
- Dietary Fiber = 0g
- Sugars = 0g
- Protein = 1g

Arugula perhaps better known as rocket can be found in most supermarkets now. Arugula makes it onto the superfoods list because it is packed with nutrients and has a very low calorie count. Two cups of arugula only add up to eight calories. I always have two cups of arugula in my salad, mixed with baby spinach and romaine lettuce. Arugula is perfect if you are on a low carbohydrate diet as two cups only add up to 1.5 g of carbohydrates. Wash arugula thoroughly to remove all of the grit and soil. Try to eat it raw as this keeps it nutrient rich. If you have to cook it then lightly steam it to use in stir fries or as a vegetable side.

Vitamin K is hard to come by naturally which makes arugula special as 2 cups will provide you with over fifty per cent of your daily needs. Vitamin K is good for your blood health and studies have shown it can slow down the advance of osteoporosis. Vitamin B in the form of folate is also in abundance in arugula, essential for pregnant women to avoid certain birth defects. Folate is also good for red blood cell health and the production of energy for the body. As arugula is quite bitter I find mixing it with baby spinach and romaine lettuce helps to tone down the bitterness and add a nice contrast of flavors. As a dressing I use balsamic vinegar so as not to add more calories.

Avocado

- 1 quarter
- Calories = 50
- Total Carbohydrates = 3g
- Cholesterol = 0g
- Sodium = 0g
- Total Fat = 5g
- Saturated Fat = 1g
- Dietary Fiber = 3g
- Sugars = 0g
- Protein = 1g

The almighty avocado fruit is one of my favorite superfoods. They are overflowing with the best omega 3's you can find in their natural state and add 20 vitamins and minerals per serving. They are one of the best alkalizing foods around and are rich in vitamin E which aids in healthy skin, lush hair and is a great anti wrinkle weapon. I eat a quarter of an avocado every day, when in season. I add them to super smoothies, dice and add to green salads and I replace butter with them as a spread. I freeze a lot of them for the off season when they are at their cheapest. Always puree them first with 1 tablespoon of lemon juice per 2 avocados. Place into sealed containers making sure to leave some space at the top, and freeze. Avocados when eaten in conjunction with other fruit and vegetables speed up the absorption of nutrients.

The quality of the fat is more important than the quantity of the fat. The fat in avocados is monounsaturated fat which is good fat our body needs. The calories in avocados are likewise good calories. A quarter of an avocado a day can help your cardiovascular system and help reduce insulin resistance. Diabetes is something we all need to watch with our unhealthy modern lifestyle.

Banana

- 1 medium size – 120g
- Calories = 100
- Total Carbohydrates = 25g
- Cholesterol = 0g
- Sodium = 0g
- Total Fat = 0g
- Saturated Fat = 0g
- Dietary Fiber = 3g
- Sugars = 14g
- Protein = 2g

I do love bananas. I often have one a day, half in a super berry and banana smoothie, and the other half in fruit salad. Bananas belong on the superfoods list for several reasons, the main reason being they are so versatile in the kitchen. Introducing your kids to superfoods is made easier when you have bananas to sweeten the deal. They have always been a staple for my super smoothies and green smoothies as the fiber really helps to bulk out the smoothie. Although the humble banana does have a lot more calories than most other superfoods at least they are the good calories your body requires. As I use bananas for sweetening a lot I can avoid using refined sugar which we all should start doing. Bananas are actually very low in saturated fats, cholesterol and sodium. Not only are they are a healthy source of dietary fiber but have plenty of vitamin c, vitamin b6, potassium and contain probiotics.

Barley

- Half a cup
- Calories – 100
- Carbohydrates – 22.7g
- Dietary Fiber – 5.6g
- Fat – 1.2g
- Protein – 2.9g
- Thiamine (Vitamin B1) – .2mg
- Riboflavin (Vitamin B2) - .1mg
- Niacin (Vitamin B3) – 4.6mg
- Pantothenic Acid (Vitamin B5) - .3mg
- Vitamin B6 - .3mg
- Folate (Vitamin B9) 23ug
- Calcium – 29mg
- Magnesium – 79mg
- Phosphorous – 221mg
- Zinc – 2.1mg

Barley is one of the oldest cultivated grains in history but only recently has started to become recognized as an important superfood. The high levels of B vitamins, good protein quantity, and high amounts of dietary fiber make this an ideal grain to add to your diet. Another important aspect of barley is the amino acid profile. Barley contains 8 separate amino acids. This amino profile helps aid in muscle recovery from exercise.

Barley is a very flexible grain product. You can use it for making a variety of bread recipes which have an amazing nutty flavor. Barley can be cooked similar to rice and used with curry dishes, a replacement for pasta, or as a side for chicken, beef, pork and fish. One of the most popular ways to use barley is to add it to your favorite soup recipes. The nutty flavor of barley adds a delightful taste to soups while dramatically increasing their nutritional profile and increase dietary fiber.

The high amount of dietary fiber is one of the biggest reasons you should consider adding barley to your diet immediately. Dietary fiber helps to reduce the risks of colon cancer, cardio vascular disease, and aids in reducing cholesterol.

What makes barley a true superfood is the powerful benefits it provides for our bodies and the ease of adding it to our diet. Barley can be consumed as a side dish, added to soups, made into pasta, or used to make delicious breads. Get started improving your health be adding a little barley to your next pot of soup and discover how easy eating better can be. Those who are gluten intolerant should avoid barley in their diet.

Barley Grass

- 100 Grams
- Calories – 251 calories
- Fat – 5g
- Protein – 29g
- Carbohydrates – 3g

- Dietary Fiber – 39g
- Vitamin C – 191mg
- Iron – 10mg
- Potassium – 4300mg
- Organic Sodium – 50mg

Barley grass is one of my essential superfoods due to the extremely high levels of dietary fiber, organic sodium, and over 30 other vitamins and minerals. Barley grass has many similar properties to fresh green spinach but is more concentrated. The amount of dietary fiber is higher and even iron, which spinach is famous for, is more concentrated in barley grass. There are two different ways I like to use barley grass. When I'm in a hurry the easiest way to get all the benefits of barley grass is to take capsules which contain barley grass powder. They are easy to take along on vacation, business trips, or to keep in the desk at the office. The other method is to drink barley grass juice. I enjoy the juice, but that is true for everyone. I'd recommend you try the juice and see if you like it. The juice provides a more powerful and natural blend of the wide range of vitamins closer to a natural state than the dried powders.

Many people who have gluten allergies express concerns about using barley grass but they have nothing really to worry about. Barley grass is harvested long before the grain head of the barley plant begin to form. Gluten is found in the grain of the barley plant, not in the grass. However there is a small chance of gluten contamination in barley grass, so if you suffer from celiacs disease, gluten intolerance or wheat intolerance I would avoid consuming barley grass.

One of the biggest benefits found in barley grass is due to the wide range of vitamins and minerals which work in concert to give you higher absorption levels. This means your body gets higher levels of benefit because the Vitamin C is present to aid in absorbing iron; the B12 is available to aid in the absorption of folic acid and so on. Barley grass may not be your most delicious superfood, but it is one of your most important.

Beans

- 1 cup cooked in water
- Calories = 235
- Total Carbohydrates = 44g
- Cholesterol = 0g
- Sodium = 0g
- Total Fat = 1g
- Saturated Fat = 0g
- Dietary Fiber = 15g
- Sugars = 4g
- Protein = 14g

Beans have been called the "poor man's meat" but now we know too much meat makes for a poor man. Over the last year I have replaced half my meat consumption with beans and as a result have lost weight and I am much healthier. As westerners we eat far too much meat and can easily replace half the protein we get from it with beans. Diabetes, heart disease and many types of cancer are connected with too much meat consumption. An average of 5-10 pounds of undigested meat sits in an adult's stomach, a breeding ground for cancer.

This is why I swapped for beans. Beans are a great low fat source of protein for your body. Mix the beans with a small portion of rice and all the amino acids are covered. The average adult needs about 50g of protein per day. One cup of beans provides nearly a third. Beans are high in folate, potassium, magnesium and iron. They contain good fats for your body and are high in soluble and insoluble fiber, B vitamins and phytonutrients.

Black Beans

- 100 grams
- Calories – 341
- Carbohydrates – 62g
- Protein – 22g
- Sugars – 2g
- Dietary Fiber – 15g
- Calcium – 12% Daily Value
- Iron – 28% Daily Value
- Folate – 111% Daily Value
- Thiamin – 60% Daily Value
- Magnesium – 43% Daily Value
- Potassium – 42% Daily Value
- Copper – 42% Daily Value
- Manganese – 53% Daily Value

You do keep a bag of black beans in your cupboard, right? This superfood is an essential for vegetarians and should be in everyone's kitchen. The amazingly high amounts of minerals, vitamins, dietary fiber, and protein make this one of the world's best superfoods. The protein contains all essential amino acids.

Most of us think of black beans as being a part of spicy Mexican dishes, since that is where we most commonly see them used. These small black beans are very versatile and can be used in a variety of recipes as a replacement for other beans and as a highly filling addition to a variety of soups. My favorite way is the more traditional method of cooking black beans by boiling them. I enjoy adding a few hot peppers to the pot to spice up the mixture and then eat them with whole wheat tortillas, corn bread, or rice.

With their high fiber content black beans are beneficial for heart and colon health. They are packed with antioxidants which can aid in improving cell health. The best news found in black beans though is the high quality protein you get with extremely low fat levels, a reasonable calorie count, and almost zero negative effects. The combination of high fiber and protein helps to slow digestion and regulate sugar levels. The overall benefits of black beans are what puts it as one of the preferred superfoods throughout South America and in many other portions of the world. Grab a bag the next time you are in the store and try these delicious beans in your diet.

Black Tea

- 100 grams (Brewed)
- Calories – 1
- Carbohydrates -0g
- Fat – 0g
- Protein – 0g

How is this possible? How can black tea be classified as a superfood when it has zero calories and almost no vitamins and minerals? The reason can be found pounding inside your chest. Black tea has been shown to play a role in reducing cardiovascular disease events. This is even true for patients with existing coronary artery disease. In a study done at Boston University it was shown that black tea reduces and even can reverse endothelial vasomotor dysfunction. That is a fancy way of saying black tea is good for your heart, but that is not all it can do for you.

Black tea contains enough caffeine to stimulate your body's metabolism slightly and has been shown to reduce appetite responses. This makes black tea an excellent drink for people who are attempting to lose weight. Black tea is also filled with antioxidants which can be beneficial in reducing cancer risk, reducing chronic disease, and even reducing the effects of aging.

Black tea has become one of my favorite beverages. I try to drink at least one cup of steaming brew per day. Most times I drink it without any sweetener, but do find it delicious with a little natural honey added. One warning about adding ingredients to your black tea is required. In a study conducted in Germany it was discovered adding milk to black tea neutralized the benefits to the heart. If you must add some color and flavor to your black tea consider a non-dairy creamer instead of one based on milk.

Black tea makes a great iced tea and can be used as the base for a variety of delicious dessert drinks. With zero calories, no fat, and great benefits to your heart you would be foolish to not enjoy a cup of black tea on a regular basis.

Blackberries

- 100 grams
- Calories – 43
- Carbohydrates – 10g
- Fat – 0g
- Protein – 1g
- Dietary Fiber – 5g
- Vitamin C – 35% Daily Value
- Vitamin K – 25% Daily Value
- Manganese – 32% Daily Value

Blackberries have become one of the superfoods I look forward to eating the most. These delicious black fruits provide your body with great amounts of vitamin C, vitamin K, and fair amount of dietary fiber. What makes them one of my favorites though is flavor. These little berries are one of the most flavorful fruits you can find. The make a great addition to a bowl of cereal, used on top of pancakes, or even on ice cream.

Blackberries have one feature which makes them a very powerful superfood. They are stuffed with antioxidants. Their antioxidant levels can aid your body in fighting off infections, reducing cancer risks, and other chronic diseases. There may not be a more delicious way to get your antioxidants on the planet.

There is another important ingredient in blackberries which is not reflected in nutrient charts either. Blackberries have high concentrations of tannin. Tannin has been shown to increase the strength of certain body tissues, gives added firmness and tightening to tissues, and helps the blood to coagulate faster for faster healing of wounds.

Imagine how much fun you can have with this superfood. Take a big bowl of tangy kefir, throw in handful of ripe blackberries, and then sit back and enjoy one of the best desserts you will ever eat which is going to give you massive amounts of nutrition and is 100% healthy for your body. How many other desserts can you say that about? Blackberries are one superfood you should rotate into your diet on a regular basis. Fresh blackberries are preferred but frozen blackberries are still delicious and nutritious, too. As one final suggestion, add blackberries to your favorite fruit salads to give them some added color and a little more zing.

Blueberries

- 100 grams
- Calories – 57
- Carbohydrates – 14g
- Fat – 2g
- Protein – 1g
- Sugars – 10g
- Dietary Fiber – 2g
- Vitamin C – 16% Daily Value
- Vitamin K – 24% Daily Value
- Manganese – 17% Daily Value

Did you remember to eat blueberries today? If not, it may because you did not eat blueberries yesterday. Blueberries are one superfood you do not want to ignore in your diet.   Recent studies have been showing indications that blueberries can aid in cognitive ability, reduce brain damage following a stroke, and may even aid in battling Alzheimer's disease. Let me ask you one more time, did you eat your blueberries today?

The element of blueberries which is receiving the most study is antioxidants. Blueberries provide a very rich source of antioxidants which can play role in heart health, brain health, and the overall health of your body. Antioxidants work to reduce the effects of free radicals on your body and to increase cell strength which helps to ward off disease and cancer. You can find many foods which have amazing levels of antioxidants, but not many which are so readily available, affordable, and enjoyable.

You may have thought adding blueberries to your cold cereals, oatmeal, pancakes, and desserts was just adding more delicious fun to your meals, but in reality you are providing yourself with added nutrition at a very low cost. Blueberries are low in calories, high in nutrition, and a top source of antioxidants.

There is one more major benefit of blueberries which most people do not like to discuss. They are a proven form of relief for both diarrhea and constipation. Blueberries add high amounts of soluble fiber to your diet which aids in proper digestion and elimination processes. When you want a fruit which can improve your memory, reduce the chances of getting sick, and regulates your digestive system, blueberries are the natural choice.

Broccoli Raw

- 1 cup or 3oz
- Calories = 30
- Total Carbohydrates = 2g
- Cholesterol = 0g

- Sodium = 0g
- Total Fat = 0g
- Saturated Fat = 0g
- Dietary Fiber = 2.5g
- Sugars = 1.5g
- Protein = 2.5g

I have never been a fan of broccoli but it is such a potent superfood that I add it to super green smoothies at least twice a week. Recent research at Johns Hopkins found compounds in broccoli that prevented tumors developing but reduced existing tumors dramatically. Broccoli is moderately anti-inflammatory and has a very low glycemic index level. It is packed with many of the vitamins including vitamin k and is a great source of copper and zinc. Broccoli is a great filler food, which fills up your stomach while being low in calories and saturated fat. Eat broccoli several times a week to boost your immune system. Being a nutrient dense food broccoli is also good for eye health.

Buckwheat
- 100 grams
- Calories – 343
- Fat – 3g
- Carbohydrates – 71g
- Dietary Fiber – 10g
- Protein – 13g
- Niacin – 35% DV
- Riboflavin – 25% DV
- Magnesium – 58% DV
- Iron – 12% DV
- Manganese – 65% DV
- Copper – 55% DV

Buckwheat is the amazing superfood which sounds like a grain but is actually a fruit seed more closely related to rhubarb and sorrels than to wheat. This is the superfood I recommend for anyone who suffers from gluten sensitivities. It can replace grain products and provide you with similar benefits to cereals which cause you problems. This grain replacement is overloaded with powerful minerals our body needs to function properly. The amounts of magnesium, manganese, copper, and iron are amazing. Magnesium helps to relax your blood vessels increasing blood flow. When paired with the cleansing action of the high amounts of dietary fiber buckwheat becomes an important superfood for heart and cardiovascular health.

Buckwheat is one of the most enjoyable superfoods to add to your diet. You can cook buckwheat to make porridge which is nutty and delicious. It can be added to a variety of foods including soups to enhance their flavor and nutrition. Buckwheat can be milled into flour which is used for baking breads, making noodles, and pasta. You may have already tried buckwheat and just assumed it was a regular wheat product. You will find buckwheat pancakes on menus in many good restaurants and is one of the tastiest ways to enjoy this superfood.

Even though buckwheat is gluten free it is not 100% free of causing allergic reactions. In rare cases people do have allergic reactions to buckwheat, so be aware to watch for symptoms the first time you sample this delicious superfood. I recommend you try buckwheat pancakes or buckwheat noodles for your first adventure with this superfood which can reduce cardiovascular disease, risk of cancer, and reduce cholesterol levels.

Cacao

- 100 grams
- Calories – 599
- Carbohydrates – 45.8g

- Dietary Fiber – 10.9g
- Fat – 42.7g
- Protein – 7.8g
- Vitamin K – 9% Daily Value
- Vitamin B12 – 5% Daily Value
- Iron – 66% Daily Value
- Magnesium – 57% Daily Value
- Copper – 88% Daily Value
- Manganese – 97% Daily Value

Is cacao really the food of gods as reported by the natives who cultivate this amazing bean, or is it just our favorite superfood? Cacao can be purchased in many different forms including raw cacao beans, raw powdered cacao, and of course our favorite method, dark chocolate. What I really enjoy about cacao in all of its forms is what is does for my mood as much as my body. Cacao includes a series of nutrients and chemicals which increase our natural levels of serotonin for a short period of time. Increased serotonin levels can cause improvement in our mood, reduce our appetite, improve sleep patterns, and aid the streamlining of other brain functions.

Raw cacao does not provide you with any higher benefits compared to processed chocolates, but it does help you avoid a few issues found with processed chocolates. Processed chocolates are high in hydrogenated oils and sugars which can increase weight and cause spikes in blood sugar levels. If you want to enjoy the highest benefits with the least side effects I recommend you try raw cacao products first, but if you cannot tolerate their flavor then look for processed products with the lowest amounts of sugars and fats possible. As an example, you can find many products which are made from 85% or more cacao solids. These products keep the health benefits high while giving you a touch of sweetness to make the cacao delicious.

Cacao is high in minerals, vitamins, and other health benefits, but for me it always comes back to how it helps my moods and helps to reduce my appetite. This is one superfood which has an important place in the kitchen.

Cashews

- 100 grams
- Calories – 553
- Fat – 44g
- Protein – 18g
- Carbohydrates – 33g
- Dietary Fiber – 3g
- Iron – 37% Daily Value
- Copper – 110% Daily Value
- Manganese – 83% Daily Value
- Phosphorous – 59% Daily Value
- Magnesium – 73% Daily Value
- Zinc – 39% Daily Value
- Vitamin K – 43% Daily Value
- Thiamin – 28% Daily Value

Have you ever thought of cashews as a superfood? It is one of the delicious nuts we usually think of as sinful since they taste great. The reality is these little nuts are packed with high quality protein which includes all the essential amino acids, are high in dietary fiber, protein, iron, zinc, and many other important minerals and vitamins. Even the high fat content is not a negative since the fat is the perfect blend which helps to battle high cholesterol and blood lipids. The only real negative in cashews is their high calorie count. You do not want to consume them in large quantities, unless you need the added energy for exercise, work, or other activities.

Cashews have become one of my favorite superfoods in the nut family due to their flavor, value, and flexibility. They taste great eaten by themselves, with yogurt, slivered into salads, and make a great addition to dozens of recipes. One of the favorite ways to use cashews is to keep a bag of dry roasted nuts in the house and then mix them with other nuts like almonds and walnuts to have a wonderful treat packed with energy and healthful benefits.

Cashews are filled with antioxidants, also. This helps to reduce your risk of cancer and increases cell membrane strength. If you do not regularly eat nuts it is time to get started. They can play a crucial role in improving heart health. How often do you have the opportunity to enjoy something delicious and have it improve your health at the same time?

Cayenne

- 5 grams
- Calories – 17
- Fat – 1g
- Carbohydrates – 3g
- Dietary Fiber – 1g
- Protein – 1g
- Vitamin A – 44% Daily Value
- Vitamin C – 7% Daily Value
- Iron – 2% Daily Value
- Vitamin E – 8% Daily Value

What makes Cayenne such a powerful superfood when you can only eat such small amounts at a time? As you will notice above the nutritional information is based on only 5 grams of cayenne pepper, or approximately 1 tablespoon. This spicy pepper packs an amazing density of vitamin A, C, E, and Iron in a very tiny serving, but that is not the reason I believe this is one of the superfoods you should not ignore. The real magic of cayenne is found in the capsaicin which produces the powerful heat which this pepper produces.

Capsaicin helps to stimulate blood flow in the body which can help overcome minor circulatory issues, provide relief for arthritis sufferers, and has even been reported to work as a mild male aphrodisiac to aid in minor cases of erectile dysfunction. This is just a start to the list of benefits provided by cayenne.

Eating cayenne pepper on a regular basis has been shown to reduce stomach issues including excess gas, cramping, and ulcers. Cayenne pepper is used as a method to reduce sinus congestion since the capsaicin causes increase mucus secretions. Cayenne pepper is even used in a powerful cleansing diet which helps to flush the body of toxins.

This is one superfood you want to use with a little caution. The powerful capsaicin levels can cause irritation and inflammation if used in high quantities. Some health food stores offer cayenne extract capsules which can give you the benefits with lower risks of uncomfortable side effects. Of course, the real fun with cayenne is to integrate it into your cooking to provide delicious, healthy, and spicy dishes you and your family can enjoy.

Chia

- 100 grams
- Calories – 490
- Carbohydrates – 43.8g
- Dietary Fiber – 37.7g
- Protein – 15.6g
- Fat – 30.8g
- Calcium – 63% Daily Value
- Phosphorous – 95% Daily Value
- Zinc – 23% Daily Value
- Manganese – 108% Daily Value

Chia seeds have become one of the most interesting superfoods to me. Chia has been grown for centuries but has largely been ignored by the west. It is now being found this food which was a staple of the Aztecs has some very promising health benefits. Chia is high in unsaturated fats with high levels of Omega-3 and Omega-6 in almost a perfect balance. These two fatty acids play an important role in reducing inflammation and helping to maintain proper cholesterol levels.

Eating chia seeds as part of your diet can help reduce spikes in your sugar levels and potentially stop diabetes. It is not a cure for current sufferers of diabetes but may reduce the risk of you getting diabetes in the future. Part of the reason the chia seed is so powerful is due to a balance between soluble and insoluble fiber which slows digestion and provides for a slower absorption of sugar into the bloodstream.

Chia seeds are high in antioxidants which may play a role in reducing the risk of certain types of cancer. Antioxidants pair with free radicals to help flush them from the body instead of free radicals causing damage to cell membranes and DNA.

Chia seeds can be eaten in a variety of ways. You can eat them roasted as a fun snack. You can grind them and add them bread recipes to add a delicious nutty flavor. You can cook them in soups, porridge, puddings, and a variety of other ways. One of the most common ways chia seeds are used by native growers is to make pinole which can be eaten alone or used in other recipes. Chia is one more superfood you can have fun adding to your pantry.

Chicken Breast Skinless

- 115g (4oz)
- Calories = 150
- Total Carbohydrates = 0g
- Cholesterol = 65mg
- Sodium = 110mg
- Total Fat = 2g

- Saturated Fat = 0g
- Dietary Fiber = 0g
- Sugars = 0g
- Protein = 23g

I had to include a few meats in the list as most people do eat meat. I personally have cut down my meat consumption to three meals a week with fish twice a week. For lunches I grill and thinly slice skinless chicken breast and turkey breast for sandwiches and salads. Remember deli meats have five times the sodium content. Skinless chicken breast is an easy source of good protein for muscle growth and tissue repair. If you work out or exercise a lot then chicken breast in meals several times a week will help with muscle fatigue. This amount will provide you with more than half of your daily needed protein. If you are dining out and watching the calories or wanting a reasonably healthy meal then order a grilled skinless chicken breast. Most restaurants carry chicken breast on their menu nowadays. The protein from chicken breasts is a complete protein which provides you with all of the needed amino acids. Chicken breast is low in sodium which is good for your blood pressure and high in selenium which is an antioxidant mineral.

Coconut Milk
- 100 grams
- Calories – 230
- Fat – 24g
- Carbohydrates – 6g
- Protein – 2g
- Iron - 9% Daily Value
- Vitamin C – 5% Daily Value

Coconut milk is another of those odd superfoods which does not show you why it is so important by looking at the nutrition tables. The real power of coconut milk and coconut oil can be found in what it does for heart health and the digestive system. The fat content, specifically medium chain fatty acids, can cause your cholesterol profile to improve. The other common use of coconut milk is to help with ulcers, stomach problems, and even kidney stones for certain types of stones.

Coconut milk can be used in a variety of fun ways. It is a common ingredient in many delicious Asian dishes ranging from entrée's to delightful frozen desserts. Coconut oil can be used as a substitute for other cooking oils and with its unique fat composition is much healthier than many other vegetable based oils. One of my favorite ways to use coconut milk is as an ingredient in shakes. You can replace use coconut milk as a sweet and milky juice to blend with ice, fruits, and other ingredients to make a refreshing dessert which is very nutritious and healthy.

Coconut milk can play an important role in helping you to lose weight, also. The same MFCA's which lead to lower cholesterol levels contribute to lower absorption of fat which can aid in better weight maintenance. If you have been seeking a natural solution to help your digestive system and reduce cholesterol then you should add both coconut oil and coconut milk to your kitchen. Use coconut oil in place of other oils and explore all the fun ways to use coconut milk in your menu. It may not be a food you want on a daily basis, but it is one you can enjoy on a regular basis.

Cranberries

- 100 grams
- Calories – 46
- Carbohydrates – 12g
- Fat – 0g
- Protein – 0g
- Dietary Fiber – 5g
- Vitamin C – 22% Daily Value

- Manganese – 18% Daily Value

Cranberries are usually only thought about during our holiday seasons which is sad. Cranberries have achieved the status of a superfood due to some amazing things this tiny tart fruit can do. Cranberries are under almost constant study for their effect on UTI (Urinary Tract Infections). The studies primarily focus on women, but can have beneficial effects for men, also.

At first it was believed the slightly acidic tangy cranberry was actually killing bacterial infections but studies are showing a much different answer. Cranberries affect the ability of bacteria to attach to the tissues found in the urinary tract which causes the bacteria to be flushed from the body. The secondary reason cranberries are highly effective is found in their high levels of antioxidants. These antioxidants help to strengthen cell membranes and reduce the ability of bacteria to attach and penetrate into the cell. This powerful duo from cranberries is highly important to women who suffer UTI problems at a much higher rate than men.

Another intriguing study on cranberries shows another reason they have achieved superfood status. Cranberry juice appears to inhibit the formation of plaque on teeth decreasing tooth decay.

My favorite way to eat cranberries is in a traditional cranberry salad with a big plate of turkey, but that is not reasonable for everyday consumption. Away from the holidays I enjoy cranberries sliced into salads, blended into shakes, and cranberry juice. The easiest way to get cranberries is in juice form but it does not give you the benefits of the dietary fiber. I recommend you try adding a few cranberries to the blender the next time you are creating your slush or shake. You will enjoy the tangy zest the cranberries add and the health benefits, too.

Cucumber

- 100 grams
- Calories – 15
- Carbohydrates – 4g
- Fat – 0g
- Protein – 1g
- Dietary Fiber – 0g
- Vitamin C – 5% Daily Value
- Vitamin K – 21% Daily Value

Cucumbers hold an interesting position in the superfood category. You may want to consider them the super filler of the family. As you can see from our nutrition chart there is nothing earth shattering about the amount of nutrients found in cucumbers. This is due in part to their extremely high water content. A cucumber is 96% water. What is the story which pushes cucumbers into the superfood category?

It starts off with all of that water content. The cucumber can play an important role in keeping your body fully hydrated. Cucumbers should be an essential food for anyone on a diet. They provide an easy to eat snack which is high in water, low in calories, and has no negative effects. You can snack on cucumbers almost endlessly and not have to worry about hurting your diet.

The next reason is what you are probably really searching for. Cucumbers are high in antioxidants but there is a bit of a catch. Many of the antioxidants are present in the skin, but the internal fruit. It is highly recommended you watch and slice your cucumbers with the peeling intact. Even if you are going to use your cucumbers in juicer include the peels. It makes a juice which is much higher in nutritional value.

My favorite way to eat cucumbers is the easiest way of all. I wash them in water. I cut them in quarters down the length of the cucumber and then eat. They are a delicious snack to crunch on while I work, play, or even drive my car. I never have to worry about excess calories and fat with the amazing snack, plus I get to increase my vitamin C intake, antioxidant levels, and hydration all at the same time.

Dark Chocolate

- 100 grams (85% Cacao Solids)
- Calories – 599
- Carbohydrates – 46g
- Dietary Fiber – 11g
- Protein – 8g
- Fat – 43g
- Iron – 66% Daily Value
- Magnesium – 57% Daily Value
- Phosphorous – 31% Daily Value
- Zinc – 22% Daily Value
- Copper – 88% Daily Value
- Manganese – 97% Daily Value

Dark chocolate may be the most sinful of all of our superfoods. Who would have believed just a few years ago that medical science would be recommending we eat any kind of chocolate as part of a healthy diet?

Dark chocolate has achieved the status of being a superfood due to the high levels of antioxidants, polyphenols, and other phytochemical combinations which are very healthy. A few of the claimed benefits of dark chocolate include reducing inflammation due to colitis, improved heart health, improved brain function, increased skin quality, and an improvement in mood.

There are a few warning which must accompany any recommendation on dark chocolate. Always seek the highest percent cacao solids you can enjoy with 75% or higher being recommended. The lower the density of cacao solids the more sugar, fats, and other unhealthy ingredients will be included. Processed chocolate can be very high in fats and sugars which leads to weight gain. Make sure you only eat dark chocolate in moderation.

The benefits of dark chocolate keep mounting with each new study completed, which is why I include dark chocolate in my diet a few times per week. I rotate between eating a small square of dark chocolate to including it in recipes. One of the most fun ways to add dark chocolate to my diet is to add it to a shake with a banana and yogurt. This is one of the most delicious shakes you can imagine. Dark chocolate can make a great addition to your cup of coffee or simmered into a wonderful hot beverage. Let your imagination run wild with ways to use dark chocolate, the superfood you love. Just do not forget to use it in moderation.

Flax Seed

- 100 grams
- Calories – 534
- Carbohydrates – 28.88g
- Dietary Fiber – 27.3g
- Fat – 42.16g
- Protein – 18.29g
- Vitamin B1 – 143% Daily Value
- Vitamin B2 – 13% Daily Value
- Vitamin B3 – 21% Daily Value
- Vitamin B5 – 20% Daily Value
- Vitamin B6 – 36% Daily Value
- Calcium – 26% Daily Value
- Iron – 44% Daily Value
- Magnesium – 110% Daily Value
- Phosphorous – 92% Daily Value
- Potassium – 17% Daily Value

- Zinc – 46% Daily Value

Flax seed is one of those superfoods which never get enough credit. Take a second look at the nutrition chart. These tiny seeds contain an unbelievable amount of B Vitamins, high amounts of important minerals, and provide good quantities of both protein and dietary fiber. Even the high fat content is a benefit since the fats are concentrated in Omega-3 and Omega-6 which aid in reducing cholesterol, heart diseases, and some studies even indicate it is beneficial in warding off Alzheimer's disease.

I believe one of the reasons flax seeds has fails to get enough credit is due to it having so many other uses. Flax seeds are not only an important superfood, but they play an important role in industry where the oil from flax seeds is used in painting processes, wood finishing, for making dyes. The other factor which has held this little seed back is the lack of great recipes for its use.

The best way to add flax seeds to your diet is to start adding them to your other dishes. They are a great addition to a bowl of oatmeal, to add into your bread recipes, can be blended into smoothies, added into soups, or as a garnish for other recipes.

My favorite way to use flax seed is adding a little to my morning cereal, in my soups, and when baking. Remember to keep your supply of flax seeds stored very carefully in airtight containers. The one negative to flax seeds is how fast they can turn bad when exposed to air. I prefer to keep mine sealed tight in an airtight container stored in my freezer. It only take a few moments to grab them out when I'm ready to cook.

Fruit Dried Organic
- 1 cup
- Calories = 250

- Total Carbohydrates = 85g
- Cholesterol = 0g
- Sodium = 0g
- Total Fat = 2g
- Saturated Fat = 1g
- Dietary Fiber = 10g
- Sugars = 45g
- Protein = 4g

You may be asking why dried fruit is included in the superfood list. You may be aware that dried fruit is high in sugar, calories and carbohydrates compared to the other superfoods. I have included dried fruit because if you need to lose weight you probably snack a lot on junk as I did when I was grossly overweight.

My worst time was evening television. I found the habit was so ingrained I needed to replace the crisps, chocolate, candy and fizzie with something else. After experimentation I found I needed something tasty and much healthier, and dried fruit became a suitable, much healthier replacement. The nutrient value of dried fruit is actually concentrated because of the dry volume. You should only buy organic dried fruit if you can, as not only are the nutrients concentrated but so are the residual pesticides in dried fruit concentrated, organic dried fruit should be pesticide free.

Dried fruits are low in sodium, fat and have no cholesterol. They are packed with nutrients and are a good way to ensure your daily intake of fruit is met. Dried fruit contains most of the vitamins and are rich in micronutrients such as potassium, magnesium, copper and zinc. Check your markets dried fruit is free from sulphur and sugar additives. Try for a dried mix of prunes, figs, dates, apricots, apple, raisins, cranberries, blueberries, peaches and banana. Add a few of the superfood nuts like almonds, cashews, brazil nuts and pistachio's to the mix and you will never reach for candy bar again.

Goji Berries

- 100 grams
- Calories – 403
- Fat – 5.8g
- Carbohydrates – 86.4g
- Dietary Fiber – 10.8
- Sugars – 75.6g
- Protein – 3.6g
- Vitamin A - 612% Daily Value
- Vitamin C – 72% Daily Value
- Calcium -29% Daily Value
- Iron – 43% Daily Value

Goji berries have been cursed with being one of the most overhyped superfoods while at the same time being one of the most important. I first became aware of goji berries because of the overwhelming marketing push going on, but that nearly pushed me away from trying them. What will change your mind is what you see in the nutrition chart above and on other factor.

Goji berries are one of the highest providers of vitamin A you are going to find in a natural food. Vitamin A is suspected of playing a major role in reducing the effects of aging and helping our bodies to utilize other nutrients more efficiently. The item which is missing from the chart above is the density of antioxidants in goji berries. These small berries, also known as wolfberries, are one of the richest sources of antioxidants in a natural form. Antioxidants play an important role in maintaining cell membrane strength and protecting our DNA from damage from free radicals. This in turn reduces our risks of cancer and many other age related diseases.

Goji berries are available in a wide variety of forms including fresh, frozen, freeze dried, powdered, in juices, and puree'. I prefer to get my goji berries in as close to original form as possible so usually choose fresh or frozen when available. Goji berries have a pleasant taste and can be used with your cereal, mixed into shakes, or in other recipes. Goji berries must be used in moderation especially if you suffer from pollen allergies. I have never experienced any problems adding goji berries to my diet. This is just one more of the important superfoods you can use to keep your antioxidant levels high to ward off cancer and other disease.

Green Tea

- 1 Cup
- Calories – 0
- Carbohydrates – 0
- Protein – 0
- Fats – 0
- Sodium – 0
- Caffeine – 24 to 40mg

How can something which has almost zero calories, carbohydrates, fats, and protein qualify as one of my favorite superfoods? Green tea has a powerful punch of antioxidants which is nearly impossible to match with any other low calorie drink. The fact that a steaming cup of green tea is completely calorie free is an even bigger benefit. Green tea gives me a boost of energy when I need to due to the reasonable amounts of caffeine. This energy boost is not accompanied by the sudden drop off often associated with sugary energy drinks which give you an immediate rush of power and then a sudden slump.

The high concentration of antioxidants in green tea teamed with the caffeine has been under intensive study in both human and animal studies and the results are very promising. There is evidence indicating consuming green tea can reduce the onset or severity of cancer, heart disease, and helps in the battle against obesity. These powerful benefits are all coming from a steaming little cup of green tea which tastes delicious and helps you relax. Can a food get any more super than that?

You can find green tea extracts and capsules you can take as supplements, but the best method of using green tea is the old fashioned way. Get out your tea pot, add your favorite green tea leaves, and let it steep. As researchers have indicated, it is currently impossible to determine if supplements made from green tea have the same benefits. All tests are currently being done on sections of the population who consume green tea by drinking it. If you do not have green tea in your home today, I suggest you head get some immediately. It is a delightful way to improve your health which you will come to enjoy as some of your best moments of the day.

Honey

- 100 grams
- Calories – 364
- Carbohydrates – 82g
- Fat – 0g
- Protein – 0g
- Dietary Fiber – 0g

Honey has the distinction of being one of the longest used superfoods, but probably not in the way you suspect. In modern times we think of honey as being that wonderful alternative to sugar which provides us with a unique sweet flavor for tea, coffee, and other uses. In historic times honey was used extensively as an antibacterial and healing salve. In recent years science has begun to uncover all of the miraculous ways honey aids in healing both used externally and when consumed.

One of the best uses of honey today is to treat the common cough. In one study it was discovered buckwheat honey was more effective than the powerful cough medicine dextromethorphan. This validates what our mothers and grandmothers have always told us. A spoonful of honey, or a cup of tea with honey, does really help our cough. This only touches on the health benefits of honey. Honey has a wide variety of trace chemicals and antioxidants which aid in healing and improving overall health.

Another common use of raw honey is to reduce allergy symptoms. Many people have discovered by eating locally produced honey they receive low doses of the pollens which cause them problems and slowly build a resistance to the allergens. This practice must be followed with great caution especially for people with strong allergic reactions.

I have found that replacing sugar with honey can improve overall health, reduce my cough, and tastes better. The antibacterial properties of honey may play a role in reducing sore throats and other conditions caused by colds, also. All I know for sure is that honey improves my life and is one of the most appreciated superfoods in my kitchen. It is the natural sweetener which can heal.

Hot Peppers

- 90g
- Calories – 27
- Carbohydrates – 6g
- Fats – 1g
- Protein – 1g
- Vitamin A – 14% Daily Value
- Vitamin C – 66% Daily Value

Hot peppers and chili peppers are a family of superfoods which provide great health benefits and an amazing taste treat. When you look at the nutritional facts of hot peppers they are not overwhelmingly impressive. The amount of Vitamin C is high, but otherwise it is a fairly empty looking profile. The magic of hot peppers is in their bite. The powerful ingredient hidden in hot peppers is capsaicin. This chemical is what gives the peppers their powerfully hot kick which we love to add to our foods.

Capsaicin does much more than just provides us with a flavorful punch. It can aid in pain reduction associated with arthritis, headaches, diabetic neuropathy, and other conditions. When you eat hot peppers it increases your circulation which can aid in reduction of many circulatory issues. There is a counter side to the heat though. You do not want to consume too many hot peppers or you may suffer from an irritated stomach or painful bowel movements as the capsaicin exits.

Adding hot peppers to your diet can aid in reducing congestion due to colds and allergies as the heat effects because increased mucus movement and an opening of sinus tissues. There are two reasons I put hot peppers down as one of my favorite superfoods. It gives me a delightful explosion of flavor and enjoyment in eating plus it stimulates my metabolism allowing me to get more done. That sensation of heat and increased circulation gets me up and moving. Hot peppers come in a wide variety of flavors and heats ranging for mild bell peppers all the way to the intense heat of habanero and other specially bred peppers which can singe your eyebrows. Hot peppers can be used to spice up salads, pizza, rice dishes, or even add them to your hamburger. Just be ready with a glass of ice water to help cool the heat.

Kale

- 100g
- Calories – 50
- Carbohydrates – 5.63
- Dietary Fiber – 2g
- Fat - 1g
- Protein – 3.3g
- Vitamin A – 308% Daily Value
- Vitamin C – 200% Daily Value
- Vitamin K – 1021% Daily Value
- Calcium – 14% Daily Value

- Potassium – 13% Daily Value
- Manganese – 39% Daily Value

Kale has to be one of the easiest superfoods for you to use and get high benefits from. Imagine having a simple green form of cabbage which tastes great in salads, soups, mixed with mashed potatoes, in stews, and hundreds of other recipes which provides you with low calories, almost zero fat and amazing quantities of vitamins and minerals. Kale is one of the true superfoods we manage to forget which is easy to add to our diet. When you look at our nutrition chart you are getting only a small sampling of the benefits of this food. There are over 20 other minerals and vitamins which kale provides in substantial quantities.

The high amounts of vitamins A, C, and K along with a high density of other antioxidants makes kale a very powerful superfood in the battle against cell membrane decay and DNA degradation which can lead to the formation of cancer. Vitamin K is a key element in our body's ability to control inflammation which can cause pain from arthritis and other conditions.

Kale is readily available in many supermarkets and health food stores and should become a staple in your kitchen. You will discover it can be used in a multitude of ways in recipes, salads, and dips to make delicious food with unbelievable health benefits. Is there any reason you would not want to enjoy a food which tastes great, is easy to cook, and relatively inexpensive? Kale qualifies as one of the best superfoods I look for in the market every time I go. It is an essential.

Kidney Beans

- 100 grams
- Calories – 337
- Carbohydrates – 61g
- Fats – 1g

- Protein – 23g
- Dietary Fiber – 15g
- Iron – 37% Daily Value
- Thiamin – 41% Daily Value
- Folate – 98% Daily Value
- Phosphorous – 41% Daily Value
- Magnesium – 34% Daily Value
- Potassium – 39% Daily Value
- Copper – 35% Daily Value
- Manganese – 56% Daily Value

Kidney beans are one of those superfoods your probably eat without even thinking about it. Whenever you enjoy a bowl of spicy chili you are getting a great source of protein, minerals, vitamins, and antioxidants all at the same time. You may be buying kidney beans and not even know it. Those cans of chili beans you buy for salads, making chili, and dips are usually made from seasoned red kidney beans.

If you take a moment and glance at our nutrition chart you can a few of the benefits to eating kidney beans, but it is not the complete story. Those 23 grams of protein comprise all of the essential amino acids making them a high quality protein source which does not require complementary foods. The high levels of fiber help you to feel full and aid in improved digestion, slowing of sugar absorption, and helps to reduce the risk of some types of cancer. Kidney beans have one other big advantage for you. They are very inexpensive. This is one of the superfoods which can help you stretch your budget while you improve your health. Canned kidney beans are usually very cheap but the dried beans are lower in price.

I enjoy using kidney beans in my soups, especially spicy soups like chili, and as an addition to my salads. The beans provide me with added protein, high nutrition, and massive amounts of antioxidants to improve my health and ward off premature aging. This is one of my essential superfoods to keep in the kitchen due to taste, versatility, and health benefits.

Kiwifruit

- 100 grams
- Calories – 61
- Fat – 1g
- Carbohydrates – 15g
- Dietary Fiber – 3g
- Sugars – 9g
- Protein – 1g
- Vitamin C – 155% Daily Value

Kiwifruit is the amazing superfood which can replace aspirin therapy in the battle against blood clots. Imagine being able to eat a couple pieces of decadently delicious fruit per day and get amazing health benefits instead of taking aspirin which can cause ulcers and other problems. Kiwifruit is one of my favorite ways to get my daily dose of vitamin C, also. It has more vitamin C than oranges and just a small amount of fruit can help you exceed your daily requirements.

Another interesting use of this superfood has been to aid in the reduction of asthma symptoms and attacks in children. In one study children eating kiwifruit or citrus fruits 5 or more times per week reduced their attacks by 44%. Imagine being able to improve your child's health dramatically by simple asking them to eat a delicious snack.

My favorite way to eat kiwifruit is fresh or in a fruit salad. Make sure you do not try to use kiwifruit in shakes, smoothies, or salads which have dairy products unless you are going to immediately consume them. Kiwifruit contains actinidin which will start to digest the milk proteins within just a few hours. For the same reason you should not use kiwifruits in gelatin based desserts either. It will start to dissolve the collagen which makes gelatin hard. These same properties make kiwifruit a great addition in another location though. Puree' kiwifruit into a blend of other ingredients to make a meat marinade which tenderizes and sweetens your favorite meats before grilling.

Kiwifruit is available in most large grocery stores and is one of the most delicious superfoods you will ever find. If you have never tried kiwifruit it is time. You will be amazed by the flavor and benefits.

Lentils

- 100 grams
- Calories – 353
- Fat – 1g
- Carbohydrates – 60g
- Dietary Fiber – 30g
- Protein – 26g
- Iron – 42% Daily Value

Why do the lowly lentils manage to qualify as a superfood? The answer can be seen in a few factors. Lentils provide a high amount of high quality protein which is only missing two essential amino acids. When the lentils are soaked in water and allowed to sprout the two missing amino acids appear giving lentils a protein value and complete protein only matched by soybeans in the plant world.

The second factor which pushes lentils into the superfood category is the high amounts of dietary fiber combined with an amazing amount of high quality energy. Lentils provide the necessary fiber to help you body flush out cholesterol and improve your cardiovascular health. The energy profile of lentils gives you energy to burn throughout the day.

Lentils are another of the very flexible superfoods. I enjoy using lentils in soups, stir fry, stews, salads, and even add them to meatloaf. Lentils have the ability to absorb flavors from other foods and become a great filling addition to almost any recipe. In the Asian world lentils are often combined with rice to add flavor and then used with curry dishes, spicy Thai recipes, sweet and sour dishes, and a variety of recipes using soy sauce.

One of my favorite ways to use lentils is to allow them to soak and sprout and then cook them in a delicious stir fry with a variety of other vegetables. With the complete protein profile of the lentil sprouts you eliminate the need for meats cutting costs and reducing fat dramatically. Lentils are also high in iron and when paired with other superfoods like kale or spinach can provide us with all the iron we require without ever taking a bite of meat. Lentils should become a staple in your kitchen you can pull out to increase the healthiness of meals and to extend your budget at the same time.

Maca Root

- 100 grams
- Calories – 325
- Protein – 14g
- Carbohydrates – 75g
- Fats – 2.2g
- Dietary Fiber – 8.5g

Why has the Maca root become known as a superfood? This intriguing food comes out of Peru where it reportedly has been used by residents for centuries to increase their libido and overcome possible sexual problems, but that is not the real story behind this food. The real story can be found in the fact this food has a very complete nutritional profile which gives a good balance of calories, dietary fiber, protein, and provides 19 of the 20 essential amino acids.

In my research I have found the claims about an increase in libido to be a highly mixed issue. In some studies it has been observed men experience an increase in sexual desire by no increase in sexual performance. The only tests which have shown any higher advantages have involved animals, not humans.

I personally do not worry about that issue. I choose the maca root as one of my favorite superfoods for other reasons. First, it is a delightful addition to my menu. The taste is a little sweet similar to sweet potatoes or other sweet roots. The maca root provides a wide range of vitamins, minerals, and antioxidants along with being a great source of dietary fiber. It makes a great addition to my diet to help reduce the risks of cancer, heart disease, and to provide all the nutrients I need for high energy. Those factors may be the reason many men and women have reported an increased libido in the first place. When you feel healthy, energized, and your body has all the nutrients you need you can perform in all aspects of your life. I enjoy eating my maca root boiled or roasted but it can be used to replace potatoes in many recipes. Give the maca root a try and see what you think for yourself.

Noni

- 1 Cup Pure Juice
- Calories – 30
- Carbohydrates – 3.4g
- Fat - <.1g
- Protein - .43g
- Dietary Fiber - <.2g
- Sugars – 1.49g
- Vitamin C – 33.65mg
- Calcium – 10.1mg

How can the Noni fruit be listed as a superfood with this very unimpressive list of nutritional benefits? Sometimes the benefits are not hidden in nutrition but are the intriguing effects of eating the fruit. The Noni fruit has been undergoing scientific investigation for helping to control diabetes. In one study a noni extract was shown to normalize glucose levels in rats.

The incredible Noni fruit appears to have a chemical composition which aids in protecting brain cells. In another study on rats damage to brain tissue was dramatically reduced when subjected to low oxygen levels. Another study shows Noni supplements and juices can aid in increasing the strength of our immune system by increasing cytokines in our body.

The most common uses for Noni juice are a little less glamorous. Natives where the fruit grows use it for treating constipation, diarrhea, and mouth sores. It is commonly recommended by local healers in to aid in the onset of cancer. All of these claims are being investigated by scientists with many claims looking promising.

This may be one of the hardest superfoods for you to enjoy. Natural noni fruit has a very pungent smell similar to dirty gym socks. The flavor is not overly pleasant either. Many people claim the fresh fruit has a flavor similar to outdated prune juice or cheese. Most users of this superfood prefer to use it as either a dried powder or in a juice blended with other fruit juices. My personal favorite is to use either the powder or juice mixed in a fresh fruit shake using bananas, mango, blueberries, or strawberries. Their sweet flavors and smells overshadow the noni fruit and I still get all the benefits.

Olive Oil

- 100 grams (Cold Pressed Extra Virgin)
- Calories – 884

- Carbohydrates – 0g
- Fat – 14g
- Protein – 0g
- Dietary Fiber – 0g
- Vitamin E – 72% Daily Value
- Vitamin K – 75% Daily Value

Cold pressed extra virgin olive oil is one superfood which is mandatory in your kitchen. It is one of those essential cooking items which anyone serious about eating properly must have. Before we get into the health benefits it is important to point out an important fact about our nutrition chart. You will not be eating 100 grams of olive oil. The real health benefits of olive oil are much more subtle. It is critical to note the benefits are from cold pressed extra virgin olive oil, not all olive oils have the same benefits.

Olive oil has one critical claim to fame which is why it must be in your kitchen. Olive oil plays an important role in decreasing heart disease when compared to other types of oils. The hydroxytyrosol in olive oil appears to protect our arteries from damage and build-up which leads to blocked arteries. Olive oil has impressive anti-inflammatory effects which provide other health benefits. Olive oil has even been shown to reduce cancer risk for a wide variety of cancers. Now, you need to ask yourself an important question. Do you really want to keep using other oils for your salad dressings and cooking when you could be improving your health?

Cold pressed extra virgin olive oil has become an essential in my kitchen. I use it to mix with vinegars, herbs, and seasonings to make marinades, dressings, and for using to lightly coat pans for frying. The added flavor from olive oil is just an added benefit which goes hand-in-hand with the great benefits to my health. Once you have started using olive oil you will find it hard to go back.

Onions

- 100 grams
- Calories – 40
- Carbohydrates – 9g
- Fat – 0g
- Protein – 1g
- Dietary Fiber – 2g
- Vitamin C – 12% Daily Value

Onions may be the most commonly used superfood in our list. They are used in recipes, eaten raw, and added as a garnish to many foods, but none of that explains why it is a superfood. Onions are not particularly high in any vitamins or minerals, but still provide some very important health benefits.

The power of onions can be traced to their high levels of antioxidants and other chemical compounds which have been reported to reduce inflammation, decrease cholesterol levels, and restrict the growth of cancer. The one which has received the most scientific investigation is the role cancer play in restricting the growth of certain cancers. Studies have shown eating onions several times per week can reduce the risks of ovarian cancer, colorectal cancer, and laryngeal cancer.

What makes onions even more important as part of your diet is the fact their antioxidant levels and benefits are not lost while cooking. When used in soups, gravies, and other recipes their powerful benefits are transferred into the surrounding foods and remain highly available. This allows you to get all the benefits by using onions just like you do today, as part of numerous recipes.

Onions are one of my key kitchen ingredients. I use onions in a wide variety of recipes but also love to eat certain varieties raw. One of my favorites is to slice onions with a bowl full of cucumber and then add a touch of vinegar and fresh ground pepper to make a duo of superfoods which taste delicious together.   If you are one of those rare people who do not enjoy onions you may want to take the time to explore. The onion family contains a wide variety of flavors and textures which can provide you with great health benefits.

Pineapples

- **1 cup raw**
- Calories = 70
- Total Carbohydrates = 18g
- Cholesterol = 0g
- Sodium = 0g
- Total Fat = 0g
- Saturated Fat = 0g
- Dietary Fiber = 2g
- Sugars = 13g
- Protein = 1g

Inflammation is at the root of all disease and as pineapple contains a lot of bromelain which not only thins blood but is anti-inflammatory as well and helps to reduce swelling, bruising and redness. Bromelain has been used to reduce pain and swelling for sufferers of arthritis. Bromelain is also beneficial for your heart and circulation as it thins the blood and reduces the chance of strokes and heart attacks. Bromelain is also good for asthmatics as it thins out the mucus in the lungs allowing for easier breathing. Bromelain also helps to break down protein and aids digestion.

But in order to gain the maximum benefit from bromelain you must eat it raw, not canned. Unfortunately most of the bromelain is located in the core of the pineapple so a fresh pineapple that you have prepared will enable you to enjoy the core as well as the remaining fruit.

Pomegranate Juice

- 100 grams
- Calories – 54
- Carbohydrates – 13g
- Sugars – 13g
- Fat – 0g
- Protein – 0g

Pomegranate juice is one of the most intriguing superfoods around. The juice is filled with antioxidants, vitamins, and minerals. The juice has been shown to aid in heart health in several different ways. The pomegranate juice has anti-clogging properties which help protect the heart from arterial blockage. The antioxidants increase cellular health including increasing cell membrane health. The stronger cell membranes help to reduce the chances of cancer, infections, and disease. Drink only pure pomegranate juice with no added sugar.

What makes pomegranate juice more impressive to most people is the wonderful flavor. It is great to drink alone or in blends with other juices. An eight ounce juice of pomegranate juice provides over half of your daily requirements for vitamin C, vitamin E, and vitamin A. I prefer to use my pomegranate juice in a green smoothie. It makes a great drink for a hot summer day. Another way I enjoy pomegranate juice is to add a few ounces to a large glass of iced tea. It provides a sweet fruity flavor to the tea.

You need to keep in mind the high sugar levels of pomegranate juice when you add it to your diet. It is not recommended for people who struggle with managing their sugar levels. If you are attempting to lose weight you should use pomegranate juice in moderation, perhaps only drinking the juice a few times per week. You can still get most of the benefits of pomegranate juice without the risk of gaining weight.

Pomegranate juice can be used as a high quality alternative to other highly nutritious juices like acai, goji, or blueberry. The powerful antioxidant effects of pomegranate juice along with the anti-clogging behavior should make it one juice you drink on a regular basis. It will improve your health in a very tasteful way.

Prunes

- 100 grams
- Calories – 240
- Carbohydrates – 64g
- Sugars – 38g
- Protein – 2g
- Fat – 0g
- Vitamin A – 16% Daily Value
- Vitamin K – 74% Daily Value

What is the first thing which pops into your mind when you hear prunes called a superfood? You are probably envisioning the well known effect of prunes ending constipation. This is just a tiny part of what prunes can do for you, but is not an item you should be concerned with. It is true prunes make an excellent laxative if you are having problems, but they do not cause problems for people who are having normal bowel function.

The second claim to superfood status for prunes comes from their high density in antioxidants. These dried plums are packed with vitamin A and K plus a wide variety of other antioxidant compounds. This helps to improve overall health and my stop the effects of aging. Antioxidant research is one of the hottest topics in food studies today with most studies showing dramatic benefits for people who consume large amounts of antioxidant rich foods.

Prunes are one of my favorite snacks. Eating a few dried plums along with a handful of almonds, cashews, or other nuts provides added energy, a well-balanced mix of nutrients, and enormous amounts of health improving antioxidants. Prunes are great to use in cooking, too. They make a great addition to sweet breads, puddings, and other sweet desserts.

If you ever have trouble with hard bowel movements or constipation prunes are the answer. They provide a natural easy to use method to correct your body's imbalances restoring you to natural bowel routines. Adding one or two prunes to your morning breakfast is a sure method to stay regular eliminating most bouts with both diarrhea and constipation. Keep a bag of prunes in your kitchen to provide you with a high-powered snack which improves your health.

Purple Sweet Potato

- 100g
- Calories – 360
- Carbohydrates – 20g
- Protein – 1.6g
- Fat - .05g
- Dietary Fiber – 3g
- Calcium – 30mg
- Potassium – 337mg
- Vitamin A – 14187 IU
- Beta Carotene – 8509mcg

The purple sweet potato has become one of my favorite superfoods for several reasons but the leading reason may be taste. These deep purple versions of sweet potatoes have a delicious sweet taste which makes them great to eat as part of any meal. You can boil, steam, bake, or roast the sweet potatoes. Steaming and boiling are the two recommended methods of cooking to enhance the nutritional benefits of this amazing superfood.

As you glance at the nutritional chart above two numbers should stand out. Purple sweet potatoes provide over 3 times the daily requirements for Vitamin A and have highly concentrated levels of beta carotene, but these two items are not what have researchers the most excited. Purple sweet potatoes are rich in cyaniding and peonidin which appear to have cancer inhibiting qualities. Their high levels of antioxidants and phenols aid in reducing the effects of aging and improving overall health.

Purple sweet potatoes have other health benefits, too. Their chemical composition provides a natural anti-inflammatory effect. Other traits include aiding in proper blood clotting, balancing blood sugar levels, and the high levels of Vitamin A and beta carotene can aid in skin tone and improve night vision for some people.

Purple sweet potatoes are becoming more common in mainstream grocery stores with each passing year, but if you do not find them there check your local health food stores and Asian markets. Purple sweet potatoes have been a staple in many Asian diets for centuries. This is one superfood you will not need to blend, disguise, or accessorize to enjoy. The purple sweet potato is delicious and nutritious all by itself.

Quinoa

- 100 grams (Uncooked)
- Calories – 368
- Carbohydrates – 64g
- Fats – 6g
- Protein – 14g
- Dietary Fiber – 7g
- Iron – 25% Daily Value
- Calcium – 5% Daily Value
- Manganese – 102% Daily Value
- Phosphorous – 46% Daily Value
- Folate – 46% Daily Value

Do you need another source of rich vegetarian protein, fiber, and energy? The tiny quinoa seeds may become one of your preferred superfoods to increase the quality of your diet and health. One of the reasons this tiny seed is marked as a superfood is due to the amino acid break down found in the protein. It provides all 9 essential amino acids which is nearly unheard of in the plant world. It can be used to supplement the amino acid profiles of other sources like rice, wheat products, and beans.

I like to eat quinoa in two different ways. You can boil a cup of quinoa similar to rice and then eat it. It has a great texture with is lighter than rice and gives you a very satisfying nutty taste. Adding a tiny touch of natural maple syrup makes an incredible breakfast treat. The second way is to use it just like rice for curry dishes, stir fry, and casseroles. It adds a unique flavor to the recipes which is a delicious alternative to rice. You can even use it in combination with rice.

In many health food stores you can find quinoa based cereal flakes which are high in nutrition and a quick alternative to cooking quinoa. Quinoa provides many other benefits other than a great protein source. It is high in antioxidants, provides a great source of dietary fiber to reduce risks of cardiovascular disease, and can even reduce migraine symptoms due to the high amounts of magnesium. Give this unique nutty seed a try. You will discover why many people consider this their favorite superfood of all.

Romaine Lettuce

- 100 grams
- Calories – 17
- Carbohydrates – 3
- Fat – 0g
- Protein – 1g
- Dietary Fiber – 2g
- Vitamin A – 174% Daily Value
- Vitamin C – 40% Daily Value
- Vitamin K – 128% Daily Value
- Folate – 34% Daily Value

Romaine lettuce makes a fabulous salad and at the same time packs a powerful nutritional treat. Romaine lettuce provides your body with amazing amounts of vitamin A, C, K, and Folate with a very low calorie count and no fat. This makes it an ideal food for people trying to lose weight. Keep in mind what you add to the lettuce, like dressings, is equally important.

The benefits from Romaine lettuce are not restricted to the vitamin content. This deep green lettuce provides you with a plentiful source of chlorophyll which has been demonstrated to improve red blood cell counts and quality. The 2 grams of dietary fiber in every 100 grams of lettuce can aid in the reduction of digestive tract problems and can help reduce cholesterol.

One of my favorite ways to eat Romaine lettuce is in a big salad. I chop up the lettuce, add a few raisins, sliced almonds or cashews, and then make a light dressing using extra virgin olive oil, vinegar, and a few herbs. The salad has a refreshing taste and provides a wide variety of flavors and health benefits.

There is one added reason Romaine lettuce should be on your table often. The high levels of antioxidants, chlorophyll, and fiber reduces the risk of both colon cancer and some forms of liver cancer. Those are both great reasons to start enjoying a delicious salad every day. Romaine lettuce may not the most exciting or exotic of our superfoods, but it does play a crucial role. It provides your body with a low calorie way to satisfy your eating urges without leaving you feeling empty.

Spaghetti Squash
- 2 cups
- Calories = 65

- Total Carbohydrates = 16g
- Cholesterol = 0g
- Sodium = 0g
- Total Fat = 1g
- Saturated Fat = 0g
- Dietary Fiber = 5g
- Sugars = 6g
- Protein = 2g

Spaghetti Squash is a superfood in its own right, but it becomes a super-superfood when you replace all of your pasta dishes with spaghetti squash. Not only does the cooked flesh of this squash look like spaghetti (hence the name) but it also makes a great spaghetti replacement. The neutral flavor of spaghetti squash lends itself perfectly to all pasta dishes but it is many times healthier for you and the nutritional value is far superior to pasta and has much less carbohydrates. Two cups of normal spaghetti would yield 400 calories with little nutritional value. I have spaghetti squash twice a week knocking 300 calories of my daily intake, each time, great for dieting. The trick to cooking spaghetti squash is to cut them in half and bake them and when done just run a fork through the flesh to create spaghetti like strands.

Spaghetti squash is enriched with vitamin c and a, calcium and dietary fiber. It also provides carotenoids which help the body fight diseases. They are a great source of several B vitamins including thiamine, folate and niacin.

Spinach
- 100 grams
- Calories – 23
- Carbohydrates – 4g
- Fats - .4g

- Protein – 3g
- Dietary Fiber – 2g
- Vitamin A – 188%
- Vitamin C – 47%
- Calcium – 10%
- Iron – 15%

Spinach has been considered a legendary superfood since the days of the Popeye cartoons, but does it really deserve the status? The answer is a loud YES. The high amounts of vitamin A, vitamin C, beta carotene, and a wide range of antioxidants and phytonutrients make spinach one of the finest superfoods you can add to your menu. Spinach has the ability to help ward off cancer, reduce inflammation in the dietary tract, and provides a rich source of calcium, iron, vitamin K, and magnesium.

One of the biggest discoveries in recent years related to the role of spinach as a superfood was found during a study of other deep green vegetables including broccoli, cabbage, Brussels sprouts, mustard greens, and others. In the study it was discovered only spinach showed a propensity to protect individuals from aggressive forms of prostate cancer. This news alone should have men lining up for a serving of spinach salad on a daily basis. It is suspected that spinach's unique blend of carotenoids is the main reason behind this discovery.

Many of us grew up with canned spinach being placed in front of us at meals and grew to dread this vegetable. It is time to overcome our imaginary distaste and try a variety of fresh green spinach recipes, dips, and soups which have an excitingly delicious flavor while providing us with a wide variety of health benefits.

Few other vegetables can claim the amazing mix of vitamins, minerals, antioxidants, carotenoids, and flavor that spinach provides. This has become one of my favorite green vegetables to use in salads to make a body empowering appetizer to my meals. Spinach should become an important part of your diet, too.

Spirulina

- 100 grams (Dried)
- Calories – 290
- Carbohydrates – 24g
- Fat – 8g
- Protein – 57g
- Sodium – 44% Daily Value
- Vitamin A – 11% Daily Value
- Vitamin C – 17% Daily Value
- Calcium – 12% Daily Value
- Iron – 158% Daily Value

Spirulina may be one of the most unusual and essential superfoods you are going to encounter. Spirulina is blue - green algae, a tiny microscopic plant. One of the most important traits of this tiny plant is the high protein content. The plant is over 60% protein making it higher in protein density than beef steaks, chicken breasts, and most traditional sources of protein. It has higher levels of iron, vitamin A, and vitamin C than most plants, also.

The high concentrations of protein become even more significant when you factor in the absorption rate. Protein from spirulina is absorbed and used by the body at a rate 4 times greater than beef. Pair this with the fact that spirulina only has 3.9 calories for each gram of protein compared to 50 calories for most meat products. This aids in keeping weight down while getting all of the protein you need.

Additionally spirulina is packed with Omega 3 acids and Gamma Linolenic Acid (GLA). These two acids can play a role in reducing cholesterol levels, aid in blood sugar control, and GLA has been shown to play an important role in the development of brain development.

One of the most amazing facts about spirulina is that it can be grown in areas which are not conducive to growing other types of foods. These blue - green algae grow heartily in waters which are two high in salt for fish to survive. You can find dried spirulina in most health food stores and in many supermarkets. A common method of using spirulina is in supplement capsules, which is my favorite method.

Split Peas

- 100 grams
- Calories – 341
- Carbohydrates – 60g
- Fats – 1g
- Protein – 25g
- Dietary Fiber – 26g
- Thiamin – 48% Daily Value
- Folate – 69% Daily Value
- Iron – 25% Daily Value
- Magnesium – 29% Daily Value
- Phosphorous – 37% Daily Value
- Potassium – 28% Daily Value
- Zinc – 20% Daily Value
- Copper – 43% Daily Value
- Manganese – 70% Daily Value

Are you ready to enjoy one of the most powerful superfoods hidden quietly in your supermarket? This is one of the superfoods which is cheap, easy to cook, and delicious. Split peas are an often overlooked item in the grocery store, which is a real tragedy. These tiny dried peas are dense in protein, dietary fiber, minerals, and vitamins. They are low in fat and sugars. Split peas provide you with a complex protein profile containing every essential amino acid.

I like to use split peas in a variety of ways. My favorite is using them in a vegetable soup. They provide the protein content I need for good health and add plenty of dietary fiber to the soup. Another place I use split peas is with my rice. I throw a handful of split peas into the cooker along with the rice and let them cook together. It adds a unique flavor and texture to the rice which tastes great with stir fry.

Split peas are very healthy for your heart for several reasons. They provide a protein source which is low in fast with zero cholesterol. They contain Omega 3 and Omega 6 fatty acids which can help control cholesterol levels. The high dietary fiber content aids in removing fat during the digestive process further reduce cholesterol levels. Split peas also aid the heart by being a great source of potassium with very low levels of sodium. Adding split peas to your pantry gives you one more alternative for protein and getting your essential minerals. They should be another essential in your home.

Sprouts

- 100 grams
- Calories – 30
- Carbohydrates – 6g
- Protein – 3g
- Fats – 0g
- Dietary Fiber – 2g
- Vitamin C – 22% Daily Value
- Vitamin K – 41% Daily Value
- Folate – 15% Daily Value

Bean sprouts are a healthy and exciting addition to your diet and can safely be categorized as another of your superfoods. In this chart we are giving you the dietary breakdown of mung bean sprouts, the most common type of sprouts eaten in the USA and throughout the Asian world. As you can see from the nutrition chart these sprouts provide a good source of protein, dietary fiber, vitamin C, vitamin K, and folate with zero fat and very low calories. Sprouts are high in water content and provide a filling addition to your meals.

Since sprouts are low in calories ad high in fiber they are a perfect addition for a person trying to lose weight. Sprouts are very filling and add very few calories to your diet. Sprouts provide a good source of protein with a wide variety of amino acids but should be combined with other foods like rice, chicken, or mushroom to provide a complete amino acid profile. Since most people use sprouts as part of a larger recipe this usually occurs without much thought.

Sprouts can be purchased in almost every grocery store but are also easy to grow on your own. You can buy the mung beans, soak them in water, and provide them with the proper combination of light and dark to have sprouts fast. Add a few sprouts to your salads, sandwiches, and stir fry to give you high doses of vitamins, protein and dietary fiber with almost no increase in calories.

Tomatoes

- 1 whole
- Calories = 25
- Total Carbohydrates = 1g
- Cholesterol = 0g
- Sodium = 0g
- Total Fat = 0g
- Saturated Fat = 0g
- Dietary Fiber = 1g
- Sugars = 2g
- Protein = 1g

It's a good thing that tomatoes make the list of superfoods as we use it so much already in our day to day diet. Did you know tomatoes were once considered poisonous as they belong to the nightshade family! In all truth tomatoes are actually super healthy and are nutrient rich. As with most red and orange fruits and vegetables, tomatoes are packed with carotenoids, namely lycopene which gives them the vibrant red coloring and also makes the tomato an anti-cancer, free radical fighting superfood. Tomatoes are extremely low in salt and refined sugars and high in dietary fiber which makes your tummy feel fuller for longer. Being cholesterol free tomatoes are a heart healthy superfood and are ideal for those watching their weight.

I add one large tomato with my superfood salad which I eat at least five times a week. The superfood salad I designed takes 200 calories off my daily limit and makes me feel fuller for longer. One decent sized tomato provides you with a third of your needed vitamin c the antioxidant champion. My superfood salad consists of one large tomato, romaine lettuce, arugula greens, spinach, grated carrot, cubed cucumber and cubed avocado. For a superfood dressing I use cold pressed virgin olive oil, balsamic vinegar and pure lemon juice quickly whisked together.

Turkey Breast

- Skinless half of a breast
- Calories = 115
- Total Carbohydrates = 20g
- Cholesterol = 0g
- Sodium = 0g
- Total Fat = 3.0g
- Saturated Fat = 0g
- Dietary Fiber = 0g
- Sugars = 0g
- Protein = 60g

Skinless Turkey breast provides plenty of protein to your diet but without a lot of fat and carbohydrates that other meats contain. The protein in skinless chicken breast is complete because it provides you with all of the amino acids your body needs daily. As far macronutrients go this one helps you build and maintain your muscle mass and keep your immune system healthy as well as helping in creating healthy blood cells. Nearly two thirds of skinless turkey breast contain monounsaturated fats which are the good fats for your heart. Skinless turkey breast is high in niacin and vitamin b6. The B vitamins help you extract energy from carbohydrates, fat and protein. The older we get the more we need to strengthen our bones and turkey is rich in phosphorus which does just that.

Walnuts

- 100 grams
- Calories – 654
- Carbohydrates – 14g
- Fat – 65g
- Protein – 15g
- Dietary Fiber – 7g
- Calcium – 10% Daily Value
- Iron – 16% Daily Value
- Thiamine – 23% Daily Value
- Folate – 25% Daily Value
- Vitamin B6 – 28% Daily Value

Walnuts come in two varieties both which have reached the level of superfood status. This nutritional chart and information covers the most common variety the English walnut which has a light colored shell and delicious nut meat. As you can see from our nutritional table the walnut has levels of several essential vitamins, minerals, and provides a great source of dietary fiber.

The fat content is what makes many people want to steer away from walnuts, but that would be a tragedy. Walnuts have a unique fat content which appear to bind with fats from other foods and actually decrease absorption and reduce heart risk. Eating walnuts at a meal which is loaded with bad fats can help to reduce the absorption of that fat and make your diet healthier.

Then we need to factor in the high levels of antioxidants packed into the meat of the walnut. It provides your body with more antioxidants per gram then most other foods you eat. I enjoy eating walnuts alone as a fun snack and cooked into many different foods. One if the easiest ways to add walnuts to your diet is to add them to salads, desserts, and other dishes which can use a slightly nutty flavor added to them.

Walnuts amazing combination of fat control, antioxidants, and high levels of protein make it a very important food for health. Buy a bag of walnuts to use in your diet and watch as your hair takes on more shine, your skin condition improves, and even mental clarity can improve. Walnuts are one of nature's most delicious snacks which provide you with great health benefits.

Wild Salmon

- 150g half fillet
- Calories = 250
- Total Carbohydrates = 0g
- Cholesterol = 100mg
- Sodium = 80mg
- Total Fat = 12g
- Saturated Fat = 2g
- Dietary Fiber = 0g
- Sugars = 0g
- Protein = 37g

Not all salmon is the same. In the Science journal in 2004 it was reported researchers discovered farmed salmon contained more than 10 times the amount of dioxins than wild salmon, attributed to the feed given farmed salmon which contains many contaminants. Remember also farmed salmon are more or less force fed to reach a prime weight much faster than their wild cousins. It makes you wonder how much nutritional value is lost as a result. If you want salmon and even canned wild salmon can't be found then purchase fresh farmed salmon and strip the skin off before cooking. As most of the dioxins are concentrated in the skin you will avoid most of the pollutants.

If fresh or frozen wild salmon is unavailable then you can settle for canned wild salmon though check the sodium levels on the can first. Wild salmon has one of the lowest mercury counts amongst different fish species.

Wild salmon is very low in saturated fats, while being high in protein and jam packed full of vitamins and minerals. Wild salmon has much higher levels of omega-3 heart healthy fatty acids than farm raised.

Wild Chinook and sockeye have the highest levels of omega-3 fat. As the body cannot manufacture omega-3 fatty acids itself wild salmon can be a good source. Omega-3 fat is essential for optimum brain functioning and body growth. If you are a meat eater you can replace two meat portions a week with wild salmon. Try to grill it or poach it rather than using processed oils for cooking. Vitamin d is rarely found in natural foods and as wild salmon is high in vitamin d you should eat it at least twice a week. Wild salmon is also rich in selenium a powerful anti-oxidant and vitamin b-12 which helps in red blood cell health.

Wheatgrass

- 1 ounce (Juice)
- Calories – 7
- Carbohydrates – 1g
- Vitamin C – 7% Daily Value

- Iron – 10% Daily Value

Why has wheatgrass become recognized as a superfood when the juice seems so low in nutrient content? The answer can be found both in history and in current times. Wheat grass juice made from the young wheat plants is filled with chlorophyll and other nutrients. All the way back in 1930 Dr. Schnabel experimented with wheat grass on his chickens to improve their health and increase their productivity. The results were phenomenal, but how does this relate to us?

The high density of chlorophyll in wheat grass stimulates red blood cell production similar to hemoglobin. This can lead to healthier blood, the ability to use oxygen more efficiently, and increases the ability of your body to transport nutrients and remove wastes from your body. This is what moves wheatgrass into the category of a superfood and has made it one of the most sought supplement juices on the market.

Wheatgrass juice alone is not highly refreshing. I prefer to use my wheatgrass juice in combination with other juices blended into green smoothies. Another big advantage wheatgrass as a supplement is the fact it is easily broken down and used by the body. It is categorized as a predigested food not requiring intense digestive processes to prepare it for absorption. It only takes a small amount of wheat grass juice to give you tremendous benefits.

Along with the chlorophyll wheatgrass is packed with antioxidants, vitamins, and minerals. It provides that extra boost to your diet to make sure you get all the nutrients you need. If you have been feeling sluggish, and low on energy, and suspect you are anemic give wheatgrass a try. You may discover it provides that energetic boost you need in a 100% natural way. There is a small chance of gluten contamination in wheatgrass, so if you suffer from celiac disease, gluten intolerance or wheat intolerance I would avoid consuming wheatgrass.

Yogurt Kefir

- 100 grams (Cow's Milk Kefir)
- Calories – 61
- Fat – 3.5g
- Protein – 3.3g
- Calcium – 120mg

Yogurt kefir is a superfood which is going to require a little bit of explanation. Technically yogurt and kefir are two separate fermented dairy products but can be combined. In most cases when we refer to yogurt kefir we are actually talking about kefir. The difference between the two is based on how they are created. Kefir is made by the addition of kefir grains to the milk which causes the formation of beneficial bacteria and active yeasts. Yogurt also contains active beneficial bacteria but not the same variety and does not have active yeast.

Yogurt kefir has the ability to rebuild your body's digestive system with the proper bacterial content for healthy digestion and better nutrient absorption. The big difference between yogurt and kefir in this respect is that kefir can implant the body with new bacterial and yeast growth, where yogurt can only enhance existing bacterial population.

Why is this bacteria and yeast so important? They can help reduce constipation, diarrhea, and provide you with increased energy. You get all of these benefits from eating a tangy delicious dairy product. The flavor of yogurt kefir is a little tangier than traditional yogurt. It can be used in smoothies, frozen treats, and mixed with fresh fruit. I am always finding new ways to use kefir in my diet and all of them are delicious. It is delicious sprinkled with nuts or crunchy cereals.

If your digestive system has been giving you problems you owe it to yourself to try this superfood. Yogurt kefir will restore the natural bacterial and yeast balance in your body which can correct numerous problems. The added benefits from increased protein, calcium, and other important vitamins and minerals are big bonuses to enjoying this delicious treat.

Conclusion

And that's 55 Superfoods, or rather 56 super healthy superfoods that you can start integrating into you daily diet. Always try and have them in their raw state as this maintains all of the nutritional value. If you can't eat them this way then always check labels for processing and added sugars and chemicals. Your feedback is important to me. Please visit my website and if you enjoyed the book and found some value in it then please leave a review at Amazon.

Katey Goodrich

Superfoods Shopping List to Print

Fresh Produce

Apples
Arugula
Avocados
Bananas
Barley grass
Beans
Black Beans
Blackberries
Blueberries
Broccoli
Cranberries
Cucumbers
Hot Peppers
Kale
Kidney Beans
Kiwifruit
Maca
Onions
Pineapples
Prunes
Purple Sweet Potatoes
Romaine Lettuce
Spaghetti Squash
Spinach
Sprouts
Tomatoes
Wheatgrass

Meat

Chicken Breast Skinless

Turkey Breast
Wild Salmon

Spices and Nuts

Almonds
Barley
Cashews
Cayenne
Walnuts

Baking

Cacao
Dark Chocolate
Extra Virgin Olive Oil
Honey

Canned Foods

Coconut Milk
Wild Salmon
Lentils

Health Foods

Acai
Barley Grass
Buckwheat
Chia
Flax seed
Fruit Dried Organic
Goji Berries

Lentils
Noni Juice
Pomegranate Juice
Quinoa
Split Peas
Spirulina
Yoghurt Kefir

Tea

Black Tea
Green Tea